ILEOSTOMY

DIET

FOR NOVICES

Enriched Recipes, Foods, Meal Plan & Procedures For Nutritional Wellness, Healthy Weight Management And More

DR. MATEO GABRIEL

DISCLAIMER

The information in this book is only meant to be used for general reading. In any way, the author and publisher do not promise or represent that the information in this work is full, correct, reliable, appropriate, or available. This includes any warranties that are expressed or implied. Because of this, you should only rely on this material at your own risk.

This book is not meant to replace professional help. If you have any questions about a subject, you should always get help from a qualified expert. The author and distributor of this book are not responsible for how the information in it is used or abused.

The author's thoughts and feelings are shown in this book. They do not necessarily represent the official policy or stance of any other person, group, employer, or business.

Any third-party material that you can get to through this book is not endorsed or backed by the author or publisher.

The information in this book is correct at the time it was published, after all possible checks. However, the author and distributor are not responsible for any loss, damage, or inconvenience that may be caused by mistakes or omissions.

TABLE OF CONTENTS

CHAPTER ONE

INTRODUCTION TO ILEOSTOMY DIET

KNOWLEDGE ABOUT ILEOSTOMY

A surgical technique called an ileostomy involves making an artificial incision in the abdominal wall through which the ileum—a section of the small intestine—is brought to the surface. Many medical disorders that impair the normal functioning of the lower gastrointestinal tract, such as congenital malformations, colorectal cancer, or inflammatory bowel illnesses, frequently call for this surgical surgery. Rerouting the passage of digestive waste to avoid the rectum and anus is the main goal of an ileostomy.

An ileostomy is essentially a practical solution for people who have difficulties with their normal intestinal functions. It involves rerouting the digestive process. The lives of those impacted by this surgical treatment may be profoundly impacted in terms of overall quality of life and medical care. Studying ileostomy's description, uses, types and the physical and psychological adaptations needed to live with one is essential to comprehending the complexities of ileostomy.

MEANING AND OBJECTIVE

An ileostomy is defined by its surgical procedure in which an abdominal incision known as a stoma is made to redirect the flow of digestive waste. Usually found on the right side of the abdomen, this stoma has a pouch attached to it to collect the feces that are expelled. This process aims to offer a workable substitute for trash removal in situations where the natural pathway is impaired or non-operational. Ileostomies are frequently used as a life-saving procedure, especially when restoration of normal bowel function by conventional methods is not possible.

Ileostomies come in a variety of forms, each designed to meet the requirements of a particular patient and certain medical issues. The three most popular varieties are the continent, loop, and end ileostomies. To eliminate waste, end ileostomy entails surgically severing the ileum's end from the remainder of the digestive tract to create a stoma. In a temporary operation known as loop ileostomy, a stoma rod is used to hold an ileum loop that has been drawn out through the abdominal wall. Continent ileostomy, sometimes referred to as a continent ileal reservoir or Kock pouch, enables the patient to hold waste until they empty it using a catheter.

GETTING USED TO HAVING AN ILEOSTOMY

Transitioning to an ileostomy is a complex procedure that goes beyond post-operative physical recuperation. People who have this surgery frequently struggle emotionally and psychologically as they adjust to the physical and daily changes. Important features of life after ileostomy include learning how to maintain and care for the stoma, choosing and fitting the right pouching device, and comprehending dietary modifications. Counseling, support groups, and medical specialists can all be quite helpful in assisting people in adjusting to the physical and emotional elements of having an ileostomy.

Understanding ileostomy entails a careful examination of its description, goals, various operation kinds, and the whole process of adapting to living with an ileostomy. Even if this surgical procedure is revolutionary, a thorough understanding is necessary to guarantee the physical and mental well-being of those dealing with the difficulties of changed gastrointestinal function.

CHAPTER TWO

AN INTRODUCTION TO ILEOSTOMY NUTRITION

NUTRITIONAL REQUIREMENTS

Because an ileostomy entails redirecting the small intestine to a hole in the abdominal wall, patients must have this treatment to maintain adequate nourishment. People must closely monitor their food choices because this rerouting of the digestive system affects how well nutrients are absorbed. Important dietary needs for ileostomy patients include maintaining electrolyte balance, staying hydrated, and having higher need for specific vitamins and minerals.

It's critical to consume enough fluids because an ileostomy may result in increased fluid loss through the stoma. Drinking enough water during the day is advised as dehydration is a possible risk. To avoid imbalances, it's important to restore electrolytes—such as salt, potassium, and magnesium—that may be lost through the stoma by food or supplements.

The significance of a well-balanced diet cannot be overstated for those who have an ileostomy, since it guarantees that they get a range of vital nutrients. A well-balanced diet promotes general health and well-being and aids in the prevention of malnutrition.

It is essential to include a range of food types to supply the essential fats, proteins, carbs, minerals, and vitamins.

It is important to keep an eye on the amount of fiber consumed because certain people may need to cut back to prevent potential problems like clogs. To support digestive health and help regulate bowel movements, it's crucial to add a variety of soluble fiber sources, such as fruits, vegetables, and oats. For the preservation and regeneration of muscles, lean proteins like chicken, fish, and tofu are essential, and a well-rounded diet should include healthy fats from sources like avocados and almonds.

COMMON DIETARY CHALLENGES

Patients with ileostomies frequently experience unique dietary issues that need to be carefully considered. The possibility of malabsorption, which can lead to vitamin deficits, is one of the main difficulties. To treat these issues, adequate dietary modifications or supplements could be required.

Some foods, especially those heavy in insoluble fiber, might irritate or cause blockages in the stoma. People need to be careful about what they eat, and they might need to try different diets to find out which foods they can tolerate and which ones they should avoid or only eat in moderation.

For ileostomy patients, it's also critical to keep an eye on their weight and nutritional status because sudden weight loss or nutritional deficiencies may indicate underlying problems. People can successfully negotiate these obstacles and make sure that their nutritional needs are satisfied through appropriate food choices and, if necessary, supplements by regularly consulting with healthcare specialists, especially dietitians.

Managing the dietary needs of people with an ileostomy requires an awareness of and attention to the nutritional requirements, a focus on the significance of a balanced diet, and the resolution of common nutritional difficulties. This method improves the quality of life for those who have an ileostomy and maintains the digestive system's normal operation while also improving general health.

CHAPTER THREE

ITEMS TO EAT WHEN FOLLOWING AN ILEOSTOMY DIET

HIGH-CALORIE FOODS

Eating a diet rich in high-calorie foods can be crucial to maintaining an ileostomy, which calls for careful monitoring of nutritional consumption. These choices make sure you get the energy you need, especially when people who have ileostomies may burn more calories because of altered digestion. High-calorie, healthful foods to consider are avocados, almonds, seeds, and olive oil. These foods include important elements like vitamins, minerals, and healthy fats in addition to a concentrated supply of calories. Including these in your diet can improve your energy and general state of well-being.

FOODS HIGH IN PROTEIN

A meal plan for an ileostomy must include protein because it is essential for tissue repair and upkeep. Eating foods high in protein supports the health of your muscles and your body as a whole. Choose lean protein sources including tofu, eggs, fish, and chicken. These choices lower the risk of discomfort around the stoma by supplying vital amino acids and being generally simpler to digest. Protein consumption should be spread out throughout the day to ensure a consistent supply of amino acids for tissue upkeep and repair.

VITAL VITAMINS AND MINERALS

Foods high in vital vitamins and minerals should be the main focus of an ileostomy diet. Making sure there is a sufficient supply of vitamins and minerals is essential since the ileum, which is in charge of absorbing numerous nutrients, may be impacted. Good sources of vital nutrients include dairy products or dairy substitutes, fresh produce, and fortified cereals. Furthermore, it can be advised to take a daily multivitamin supplement to address any potential dietary gaps. Blood tests can be used to regularly evaluate nutrient levels, which can assist in individualized diets and guarantee maximum health.

FIBER-FRIENDLY OPTIONS

Although a high-fiber diet is frequently advised for digestive health, those who have an ileostomy must use caution when consuming fiber. For those who have an ileostomy, too much fiber may cause problems due to obstructions or excessive stool production. On the other hand, it may be advantageous to include fiber-friendly options that are low in insoluble fiber.

Choose cooked veggies, peeled fruits, and sources of soluble fiber like psyllium husk and oats. In addition to improving digestive comfort, these choices help maintain regularity in the bowel without irritating the area surrounding the stoma.

Maintaining an ileostomy necessitates a careful and balanced diet. Eating foods strong in protein promotes tissue regeneration and overall bodily function while consuming high-calorie selections guarantees that energy needs are satisfied. Maintaining optimal health requires essential vitamins and minerals, and eating a diet high in fiber can help to promote digestive comfort without raising the risk of issues.

Under the direction of medical professionals, customizing the ileostomy diet to a patient's preferences and requirements can improve their general health and quality of life.

CHAPTER FOUR

THINGS NOT TO EAT WHEN HAVING AN ILEOSTOMY

HIGH-FIBRE MEALS

People who have an ileostomy are often recommended to reduce their intake of high-fiber meals. Food fiber is an important part of a balanced diet, but because it can irritate or cause blockages in the digestive tract, it can be difficult for those who have an ileostomy. Whole grains, nuts, seeds, and raw fruits and vegetables are examples of foods high in fiber that may not be well tolerated since they might cause increased stool production and possibly pain. Ileostomy patients must closely collaborate with their doctors or nutritionists to ascertain their particular fiber tolerance levels and, if necessary, reintroduce fiber into their diets gradually.

GAS-GENERATING EATS

Foods that cause gas can also be harmful to ileostomy patients. Some meals can cause the digestive tract to produce more gas, including cabbage, beans, lentils, and carbonated drinks. Overeating can cause discomfort and bloating, and it can also affect how well the ileostomy pouch works. To reduce the risk of complications, it is recommended that people who have an ileostomy identify particular meals that cause gas and limit their consumption of those items. Furthermore, eating slowly, avoiding straw drinking, and thoroughly digesting food can all help minimize the amount of extra air that is ingested, which can lessen the pain associated with gas.

UNHEALTHY FATS AND OILS

Individuals who have an ileostomy may need to closely monitor their intake of problematic fats and oils. Although lipids are a necessary component of a healthy diet, some fats might cause loose stools or increased feces production, which can be problematic for people who have ileostomies. Fried foods and fatty meat cuts are examples of foods high in saturated fats that may be more difficult to digest and cause problems with stool consistency. Moderate consumption of healthy fats, like those in avocados, olive oil, and fatty fish, is advised. Individuals with an ileostomy can make educated decisions regarding their fat intake by speaking with a dietician or healthcare expert, taking into account their individual needs and tolerances.

Controlling the diet while having an ileostomy necessitates giving serious thought to meals high in fiber, foods that cause gas, and unhealthy fats and oils.

CHAPTER FIVE

MEAL PREPARATION AND PORTION MANAGEMENT

MAKING WELL-COMPOSED MEALS

An essential component of efficient meal planning and portion control is preparing balanced meals. A well-balanced diet generally consists of a mix of micronutrients like vitamins and minerals and macronutrients like proteins, fats, and carbohydrates. This guarantees that the body gets a wide variety of nutrients that are necessary for its best possible functioning. Meal planning should take into account each person's unique dietary requirements, preferences, and any particular health objectives.

The idea of preparing balanced meals in the context of meal planning entails choosing a range of foods from various food groups. For instance, adding whole grains, lean meats, fruits, veggies, and healthy fats in the right amounts can make a meal more balanced and nourishing. This strategy promotes general health, helps sustain consistent energy levels, and may help with weight control.

CONCISE SNACKING

Another essential element of sensible portion control and meal planning is smart snacking. By bridging the gap between meals, snacks can help avoid overeating during main meals and excessive hunger. Selecting nutrient-dense snacks that support overall dietary objectives is crucial, though. Snacking on foods high in protein, fiber, and good fats will help you feel fuller and have energy for longer.

To prevent consuming too many calories, people should consider portion sizes while organizing their snack menus. Controlling portion sizes is essential for controlling weight and avoiding calorie overconsumption. One useful tactic for managing portions is to divide larger snacks into smaller pieces or to proportion them.

A healthy snacking schedule can also be achieved by being aware of hunger signs and eating thoughtfully.

Portion size management becomes even more crucial for those who have an ileostomy. An ileostomy necessitates dietary modifications since it entails the surgical construction of a hole in the abdominal wall through which the small intestine is brought to the surface. Changes in digestion and nutrient absorption may occur in ileostomy patients, necessitating adjustments to meal selections and portion levels.

PORTION SIZES FOR PATIENTS WITH ILEOSTOMIES

For ileostomy patients, portion sizes should emphasize meals that are easy to digest and easy on the digestive tract. Frequent little meals can help avoid overtaxing the digestive system. It is imperative to collaborate closely with healthcare professionals, such as dietitians and providers, to customize meal plans to meet the specific needs of each individual and address any particular issues about the digestion and absorption of nutrients.

Good meal planning and portion control entail preparing meals that are well-balanced and include a range of nutrients, selecting wisely for snacks, and adjusting portion sizes to suit each person's needs, including those of ileostomy patients. These ideas promote weight control, enhance general health, and guarantee that dietary needs are satisfied sustainably and conscientiously.

CHAPTER SIX

ILEOSTOMY AND HYDRATION

THE NEED FOR HYDRATION

Staying hydrated is essential for preserving general health and well-being, and it's even more important for those who have an ileostomy. Many physiological processes, such as digestion, nutrition absorption, temperature regulation, and waste removal, depend on adequate hydration. Because of the changes to their digestive system, people who have an ileostomy find it even more important to stay properly hydrated.

People who have an ileostomy must stay hydrated to avoid dehydration, which can happen due to the increased fluid loss brought on by the stoma. Bypassing the large intestine, the ileostomy directs the flow of waste materials and digestive juices from the small intestine to the surface of the abdomen. Because of this, vital fluids and electrolytes are lost more quickly, therefore it's critical for people who have an ileostomy to pay close attention to their fluid intake.

DRINKS TO HYDRATE

Drinking hydration-promoting beverages is essential to helping people with ileostomies stay as hydrated as possible.

The most common and organic option for preserving fluid balance is water. It is necessary to keep the body's systems operating properly and to prevent dehydration. Still, additional hydration choices including diluted fruit juices, herbal teas, and clear broths can help increase total fluid intake.

When thinking about hydration drinks for those who have an ileostomy, there are a few things to keep in mind. Drinks with a lot of sugar and caffeine should be avoided as they may cause the stoma to produce more fluid than usual. Furthermore, alcohol might dehydrate you, so you should restrict how much of it you consume.

Maintaining the body's electrolyte balance, which may be hampered in people with ileostomies, can be especially helped by balancing water consumption with electrolyte-rich liquids.

TRACKING FLUID CONSUMPTION

One of the most important aspects of ensuring proper hydration for people with ileostomies is monitoring fluid intake. Keeping a regular tab on the quantity and kinds of fluids ingested might give important information about a person's specific hydration requirements. Adjustments may be required to provide enough hydration due to factors that influence fluid requirements, including climate, physical activity, and general health. Medical practitioners frequently suggest a daily fluid consumption goal based on the unique requirements of each patient, taking age, weight, and medical history into consideration.

Those who have an ileostomy should be aware of symptoms of dehydration, such as increased thirst, dark urine, weariness, and dizziness. These symptoms should be treated right away because they might point to a deficiency in fluid intake. In addition to preventing dehydration, maintaining optimal general health, and promoting the regular operation of the urinary and digestive systems all depend on monitoring fluid intake.

Selecting appropriate hydrating beverages, being aware of the significance of being hydrated, and keeping a close eye on fluid consumption are all essential components of providing care for people with ileostomies. People who prioritize their hydration can reduce the dangers of fluid loss, improve their general health, and improve the efficiency of their digestive and urinary systems.

CHAPTER SEVEN

HEALTHY WEIGHT OBJECTIVES

MANAGING WEIGHT WITH AN ILEOSTOMY

Keeping an ileostomy at a healthy weight is an essential part of overall health for those who have had ostomy surgery. Achieving healthy weight goals is essential to maintaining the best possible physical and mental health. While the precise weight goals may change depending on the circumstances, age, gender, and weight before surgery should all be taken into account. Establishing reasonable and attainable weight goals is crucial for reducing needless stress and fostering a positive body image.

TECHNIQUES FOR RETAINING WEIGHT

Eating a healthy, well-balanced diet is one of the main tactics for maintaining weight when having an ileostomy. The secret to supplying these nutrients is to include a range of fruits, vegetables, lean meats, and whole grains. Maintaining proper hydration is particularly essential since people who have an ileostomy may be more prone to dehydration as a result of increased fluid loss. Eating smaller, more frequent meals throughout the day and keeping an eye on portion sizes might help control digestion and avoid pain.

Another essential part of controlling weight with an ileostomy is engaging in regular physical activity. Moderate physical activity, such as swimming, walking, or mild aerobics, helps maintain a healthy weight and improves cardiovascular health in general. Speak with a healthcare provider before beginning any exercise program to be sure the exercises selected are safe and appropriate for your situation.

TAKING CARE OF WEIGHT ISSUES

When dealing with weight issues, a comprehensive strategy that takes into account one's mental and physical health is necessary. People who have an ileostomy may experience particular difficulties with their self-esteem and body image. Navigating these emotional components can be greatly aided by seeking support from mental health experts, ostomy support groups, or healthcare professionals. Maintaining open lines of contact with medical professionals facilitates the resolution of any particular issues about weight fluctuations and ensures that the management plan can be modified as necessary.

It is crucial to understand that managing weight while living with an ileostomy is a unique experience, and what works for one person might not work for another. It's critical to schedule routine check-ups with medical professionals, such as nutritionists and stoma care nurses, to track weight fluctuations and modify the management plan as needed.

CHAPTER EIGHT

PARTICULAR ATTENTION TO PATIENTS WITH ILEOSTOMIES

TAKING AN ILEOSTOMY ON A TRIP

Ileostomy-related travel has special considerations that must be carefully planned for to guarantee a hassle-free and enjoyable vacation. Having a sufficient supply of ostomy supplies, such as pouches, adhesive items, and cleaning supplies, is important. To accommodate for unforeseen circumstances or delays, it is advised to bring twice as much as would be required for the duration of the trip.

Keeping supplies in a carry-on bag also guarantees accessibility when traveling, lowering the possibility of loss or damage.

Those who have an ileostomy should inform airline personnel of their medical condition when traveling to obtain the appropriate accommodations. This preemptive strategy can assist in resolving worries about security inspections and possible problems with ostomy supplies. To have a more comfortable travel experience, it is also crucial to find out if airports and other destinations provide ostomy-friendly amenities.

GETTING TOGETHER AND EATING OUT

While going out to eat and socializing might occasionally cause anxiety for those who have an ileostomy, these activities can still be enjoyable with the right planning and awareness. Open contact with friends and acquaintances helps ease any possible uneasiness since other people's compassion and understanding can help people feel more at ease in social circumstances. Eating out can be made more enjoyable by choosing foods that are less likely to create issues, such as readily digesting alternatives.

Furthermore, it can be helpful to let restaurant staff know about food limitations associated with ileostomy. This guarantees that chefs can make the required arrangements and are informed of any special demands. Selecting foods that are softer and well-cooked may be better because they are easier on the digestive tract. To properly control digestion, it's also essential to drink enough water and eat smaller, more frequently spaced meals.

MANAGING NUTRITIONAL LIMITATIONS

Living with an ileostomy requires adjusting to dietary restrictions because some foods can affect stoma function and general health. People should collaborate closely with medical specialists, such as nutritionists or ostomy nurses, to create a customized eating plan that suits their requirements and preferences. Potential issues can be avoided by being aware of which foods are better tolerated and which ones should be eaten in moderation.

For general health, it is imperative to have a balanced diet that contains an adequate intake of nutrients. Because increased fluid output might result in dehydration, people with ileostomies may need to monitor their fluid and electrolyte balance. Maintaining an eye on how various meals affect the consistency of feces and modifying one's diet accordingly can help promote better digestive health and

Ileostomy patients need to take extra care in several areas of daily living, such as traveling, interacting with others, and adhering to dietary restrictions. Individuals who have an ileostomy can confidently handle these situations by being proactive and aware, which will ultimately lead to a comfortable and meaningful life.

CHAPTER NINE
MEAL IDEAS AND RECIPES
MORNING MEAL

Breakfast is frequently regarded as the most significant meal of the day since it gives you the energy you need to start the day. Usually, a balanced breakfast consists of a mix of healthy fats, proteins, and carbohydrates. For complex carbs, whole-grain cereals, oatmeal, or whole-wheat toast are popular choices. For protein, they go well with eggs, yogurt, or nut butter. Vital vitamins and minerals are added by fresh fruits and vegetables. Smoothies can include a wide range of ingredients, such as fruits, vegetables, and protein sources, making them an adaptable option.

Pancakes, waffles, or French toast can be a great breakfast option for individuals who have a sweet craving. To increase nutritional content, try experimenting with healthier substitutes like almond or whole-grain flour. Fresh berries, Greek yogurt, or a honey drizzle are examples of toppings that can enhance flavor and provide nutritional value.

LUNCHTIME

Lunch is an important midday meal that needs to balance energy production and hunger satisfaction. With their assortment of lush greens, veggies, lean proteins like grilled chicken or tofu, and dressings to choose from, salads are a well-liked and adaptable lunch choice. With countless possible food combinations, whole-grain bread and sandwich wraps offer a lunch alternative that's both portable and adaptable.

Comforting and nourishing, warm alternatives like soups or grain bowls include lean proteins, a variety of veggies, and grains like brown rice or quinoa. A well-prepared supper's leftovers might also be a simple and quick lunch choice.

SUPPER

Dinner is sometimes regarded as the primary meal of the day and offers the chance to have a varied and fulfilling gastronomic experience. A nutritious dinner is made up of lean proteins like fish, chicken, or tofu, as well as whole grains and a variety of veggies. Cooking techniques like grilling, baking, or roasting preserve food's nutritious content while boosting flavor.

Plant-based and vegetarian choices are becoming more and more popular; vegetable stir-fries, lentil-based curries, and roasted vegetable medleys are some of the mainstays. To keep a healthy balance, it's critical to pay attention to portion control and stay away from rich, heavy sauces.

A side salad or some cooked veggies gives the meal more nutrients and freshness.

DESSERTS AND SNACKS

Between meals, snacks are essential for sustaining energy levels. Nutrient-dense snacks, such as nuts, seeds, or Greek yogurt paired with fruit, offer a filling and nutritious choice. Whole-grain crackers, a modest portion of cheese, or vegetable sticks with hummus can all be delicious options.

Desserts can be enjoyed in moderation even though they are sometimes linked to gluttony. Yogurt parfaits, dark chocolate with almonds, and fruit salads are healthier dessert alternatives. Recipes for traditional desserts can be made guilt-free by using whole-grain flour, adding fruits, and replacing refined sugars with natural sweeteners. Indulging in moderation while making thoughtful decisions guarantees that even indulgences have a favorable impact on general health.

CHAPTER TEN

SOLVING TYPICAL DIETARY PROBLEMS

MANAGING DIARRHEA

A frequent digestive problem, diarrhea can be brought on by several things, such as food intolerances, bacterial or viral infections, or certain drugs. It's critical to concentrate on rehydrating and making dietary changes when dealing with diarrhea. Since the body loses vital fluids during episodes, staying hydrated is crucial to managing diarrhea. Drinking plenty of water, electrolyte-rich beverages, and oral rehydration treatments can help replenish lost fluids and prevent dehydration.

In terms of dietary adjustments, opting for a bland and easily digestible diet is often recommended. T A popular diet is the BRAT diet, which consists of toast, applesauce, rice, and bananas. These foods are gentle on the digestive system and can help solidify stools. Additionally, avoiding greasy, spicy, and high-fiber foods during bouts of diarrhea can aid in reducing irritation to the digestive tract. Probiotics, found in yogurt or supplements, may also be beneficial in restoring a healthy balance of gut bacteria.

COMBATTING DEHYDRATION

Dehydration is a serious concern that can arise from various factors, including illness, excessive heat, or inadequate fluid intake. Adequate hydration is essential for overall health, and dehydration can lead to a range of issues, including dizziness, fatigue, and, in severe cases, organ failure. To combat dehydration, it is crucial to prioritize fluid intake.

Water is the primary and most effective choice for hydration. Consuming water throughout the day, especially during hot weather or physical activity, helps maintain the body's fluid balance. Electrolyte-rich beverages, such as sports drinks or coconut water, can be beneficial in replenishing electrolytes lost through sweat. It's important to be mindful of caffeine and alcohol consumption, as these substances can contribute to dehydration.

In addition to fluid intake, consuming water-rich foods, such as fruits and vegetables, can contribute to overall hydration. Monitoring urine color is a simple yet effective way to assess hydration levels; a pale yellow color indicates adequate hydration, while dark yellow or amber may signal dehydration.

NUTRIENT DEFICIENCY CONCERNS

Nutrient deficiencies can arise from various factors, including poor dietary choices, certain medical conditions, or inadequate absorption of nutrients. Common nutrient deficiencies include those of vitamins D, B12, iron, and calcium. Identifying and addressing these deficiencies is crucial for maintaining overall health and preventing long-term complications.

A balanced and varied diet is fundamental in preventing nutrient deficiencies. Incorporating a diverse range of fruits, vegetables, whole grains, lean proteins, and dairy or dairy alternatives can help ensure an adequate intake of essential nutrients. In cases where dietary adjustments may not be sufficient, supplements may be recommended under the guidance of a healthcare professional.

Regular monitoring of nutrient levels through blood tests can provide valuable insights into potential deficiencies. Symptoms such as fatigue, weakness, and changes in skin, hair, or nails can also serve as indicators of nutrient deficiencies.